This book was compiled by Daniel Melehi
with the A.I assistance of Inventabot

<u>Dedication</u>

I hope this helps all of my wonderful
readers achieve all their goals in their
business. And I would like to thank my
wonderful wife for all of her continued
support in all my ventures.

©Daniel Melehi

May 7 2023

Table of Contents

Chapter 1: What is Brain Fog?

Brain fog is a term used to describe the feeling of a clouded or hazy mental state, often accompanied by difficulty concentrating or remembering information. It can manifest as a sense of mental exhaustion, slow thinking, or the inability to focus. Brain fog can be frustrating and debilitating, often leading to a decrease in productivity, increased stress and anxiety, and a reduced quality of life. There are many potential causes of brain fog, ranging from stress and lack of sleep to medical conditions such as depression and anxiety. In some cases, brain fog may be a side effect of medication or a symptom of an underlying health condition. It's important to recognize the symptoms of brain fog so you can take steps to manage your condition and improve your overall quality of life. Some common symptoms include difficulty concentrating, forgetfulness, decreased alertness, and confusion. If you're experiencing any of these symptoms, it's important to speak with your healthcare provider for an accurate diagnosis and appropriate treatment plan. In the following chapters, we'll explore the various causes of brain fog, the symptoms associated with the condition, and potential coping strategies for managing this frustrating and challenging condition.

Chapter 1: What is Brain Fog?

Brain Fog is a condition that affects an individual's mental state. It is characterized by a feeling of confusion and a lack of mental clarity. Sometimes known as "brain fatigue," or "clouding of consciousness," brain fog can have a profound effect on a person's quality of life and their ability to perform daily tasks. Brain Fog is not a medical term but is a common symptom of a range of conditions and diseases. It is often associated with autoimmune disorders, chronic fatigue syndrome, fibromyalgia, and neurological disorders such as multiple sclerosis and Alzheimer's disease. Although brain fog can affect people of all ages, it is most commonly reported by older adults. Women who are pregnant or going through menopause may also experience brain fog due to hormonal changes. The symptoms of brain fog can vary, but most people report feeling mentally tired, forgetful, and easily distracted. They may find it difficult to concentrate or have trouble processing information. Some individuals may struggle to find the right words when speaking or writing. While brain fog can be frustrating, there are coping strategies and treatments that can help. It's important to seek medical attention if symptoms persist or worsen, as underlying medical conditions may need to be addressed. Through education and awareness, individuals can better understand brain fog, its causes, and how to manage it effectively.

Chapter 2: Causes of Brain Fog

Brain fog can be caused by a variety of factors, including medical conditions, lifestyle choices, and environmental factors. Identifying the cause of brain fog is an important step in finding effective coping strategies. Here are some of the most common causes of brain fog:

MEDICAL CONDITIONS

Medical conditions that affect the brain or other parts of the body can cause brain fog. Some of the most common medical causes of brain fog include:

1. Chronic Fatigue Syndrome

Chronic fatigue syndrome (CFS) is a condition that causes persistent fatigue that is not relieved by rest. People with CFS often experience brain fog as well as other cognitive symptoms such as difficulty with concentration and memory.

2. Fibromyalgia

Fibromyalgia is a chronic pain condition that can also cause brain fog. Like CFS, fibromyalgia is often accompanied by cognitive symptoms such as difficulty with memory and concentration.

3. Thyroid Disorders

Thyroid disorders such as hypothyroidism and hyperthyroidism can cause brain fog. These conditions affect the thyroid gland, which is responsible for regulating metabolism. When the thyroid gland is not functioning properly, it can lead to a variety of symptoms including brain fog.

4. Sleep Disorders

Sleep disorders such as sleep apnea and insomnia can cause brain fog. These conditions interfere with the quality of sleep, which can lead to cognitive symptoms such as difficulty with concentration and memory.

LIFESTYLE FACTORS

In addition to medical conditions, lifestyle factors can also contribute to brain fog. Some of the most common lifestyle factors that cause brain fog include:

1. Poor Diet

A poor diet that is high in processed foods and low in nutrients can cause brain fog. Nutrients such as vitamins B12 and D, omega-3 fatty acids, and antioxidants are essential for brain health, and a lack of these nutrients can lead to cognitive symptoms such as brain fog.

2. Dehydration

Dehydration can also cause brain fog. When the body is dehydrated, it can lead to a variety of symptoms including difficulty with concentration and memory.

3. Sedentary Lifestyle

A sedentary lifestyle can contribute to brain fog. Exercise is important for brain health, as it helps to increase blood flow and oxygen to the brain. A lack of exercise can lead to cognitive symptoms such as difficulty with concentration and memory.

ENVIRONMENTAL FACTORS

Environmental factors can also contribute to brain fog. Here are some of the most common environmental factors that cause brain fog:

1. Toxins

Toxins such as heavy metals, pesticides, and chemicals can cause brain fog. These toxins can build up in the body over time and lead to cognitive symptoms such as difficulty with concentration and memory.

2. Stress

Stress can also cause brain fog. When we are under stress, our bodies release hormones such as cortisol, which can affect brain function. Chronic stress can lead to cognitive symptoms such as difficulty with concentration and memory.

3. Poor Air Quality

Poor air quality can contribute to brain fog. Polluted air can contain toxins that can affect brain function, and a lack of fresh air can lead to cognitive symptoms such as difficulty with concentration and memory. Identifying the cause of brain fog can be a complex process, and it may involve working with a healthcare professional.

Once the cause has been identified, however, it becomes easier to find effective coping strategies.

Chapter 3: Symptoms of Brain Fog

When it comes to brain fog, the symptoms can be frustrating and challenging to deal with. Brain fog is not an official medical diagnosis, but it is a commonly used term to describe a collection of cognitive symptoms that can feel like a clouded mental state. One of the most prominent symptoms of brain fog is difficulty concentrating. This can manifest as the inability to focus on tasks, difficulty remembering things, or trouble with completing familiar activities, like cooking or cleaning. Another symptom of brain fog is mental fatigue, which can present as a lack of motivation and energy. When experiencing mental fatigue, one may have difficulty keeping up with their daily responsibilities or feeling like everything is just too overwhelming. For some, brain fog can also cause confusion, forgetfulness, and trouble with decision-making. One may struggle to make decisions and feel indecisive, or they may forget important appointments and dates. In addition to the symptoms above, some people with brain fog may experience other cognitive symptoms such as:

Mood changes:

Brain fog can cause irritability, anxiety, depression, and other mood changes.

Physical symptoms:

Headaches, dizziness, muscle weakness, and sleep disturbance can all be signs of brain fog.

Speech difficulties:

Difficulty finding words or forming sentences can be a symptom of brain fog. If you're experiencing any of these symptoms, it can be helpful to track them and discuss them with a healthcare professional. Understanding the symptoms of brain fog is an important first step in managing them effectively. In the next chapter, we'll dive deeper into the causes of brain fog to help shed light on why you might be experiencing these symptoms.

Chapter 4: Understanding Cognitive Dysfunction

Cognitive dysfunction, also known as brain fog, is a condition that can affect individuals of all ages. This condition can be caused by a variety of factors including stress, sleep deprivation, and medical conditions such as anxiety and depression. Cognitive dysfunction can manifest in a variety of ways, such as difficulty concentrating, forgetting things, and difficulty with decision-making. It can also cause confusion, disorientation, and a feeling of mental exhaustion.

WHAT IS COGNITIVE DYSFUNCTION?

Cognitive dysfunction is a term used to describe a range of cognitive deficits that can impact an individual's daily life. This condition can make it difficult for people to complete simple tasks, affecting their work performance, relationships, and daily living activities.

CAUSES OF COGNITIVE DYSFUNCTION

There are several causes of cognitive dysfunction, including:

Medical Conditions

Medical conditions such as anxiety, depression, chronic fatigue syndrome, and hypothyroidism can cause cognitive dysfunction. Other medical conditions such as Multiple Sclerosis, Parkinson's Disease, and Alzheimer's can also cause cognitive dysfunction.

Medications

Certain medications such as chemotherapy drugs, anti-anxiety medications, and opioids can cause cognitive dysfunction.

Sleep Deprivation

Prolonged sleep deprivation can cause cognitive dysfunction. Sleep is essential for the brain to function optimally. Without enough sleep, the brain may not be able to process information effectively.

Stress

Stressful life events can lead to cognitive dysfunction. Stress can cause an increase in the level of the stress hormone cortisol, which can affect cognitive function.

SYMPTOMS OF COGNITIVE DYSFUNCTION

Cognitive dysfunction can manifest in several ways, such as:

Difficulty Concentrating

Difficulty concentrating is a common symptom of cognitive dysfunction. Individuals with cognitive dysfunction may find it challenging to focus on tasks and may get easily distracted.

Forgetfulness

Memory problems are also common among people with cognitive dysfunction. They may forget important details or may find it difficult to remember things they have learned.

Difficulty with Decision-Making

It may be challenging for people with cognitive dysfunction to make decisions at times.

Confusion

Cognitive dysfunction can cause confusion, leading to difficulty understanding or remembering information.

Disorientation

Disorientation is another common symptom of cognitive dysfunction. Individuals may feel lost or confused about their surroundings.

Mental Exhaustion

People experiencing cognitive dysfunction may experience a feeling of mental exhaustion even after doing small tasks. Understanding cognitive dysfunction's causes and symptoms is crucial because it can impact an individual's daily life. It is important to seek treatment if you experience cognitive dysfunction to help restore your cognitive function and improve your quality of life.

Chapter 5: How Stress Affects the Brain

Stress is an inevitable part of everyday life. However, when stress levels are consistently high, it can have a detrimental effect on our overall health, including our brain function. In this chapter, we will explore the impact of stress on the brain and how it contributes to brain fog.

THE FIGHT OR FLIGHT RESPONSE

When our body perceives a threat, whether it be physical or emotional, it activates a physiological response known as the fight or flight response. This response triggers the release of hormones, including adrenaline and cortisol, to prepare the body for action.

While this response can be essential in life-threatening situations, prolonged exposure to stress can have adverse effects on the brain. High levels of cortisol can damage brain cells in the hippocampus, the area responsible for memory and learning. This damage can lead to cognitive impairment, including brain fog.

CHRONIC STRESS AND INFLAMMATION

Chronic stress can also contribute to inflammation in the brain, which can exacerbate cognitive dysfunction. Long-term stress can compromise the integrity of the blood-brain barrier, which can lead to an influx of pro-inflammatory molecules in the brain. Inflammation can also contribute to the breakdown of communication between brain cells, affecting memory, concentration, and overall cognitive function. This chronic inflammation is a common link between many neurological disorders, including Alzheimer's disease and multiple sclerosis.

MANAGING STRESS FOR BETTER BRAIN HEALTH

It's essential to manage stress levels to maintain optimal brain function. Some strategies to reduce stress and promote brain health include regular exercise, practicing mindfulness and meditation, getting adequate sleep, and avoiding excessive alcohol and caffeine consumption. Additionally, engaging in activities that promote relaxation and self-care can help reduce stress and improve brain function. These activities can include spending time with loved ones, engaging in hobbies or creative endeavors, and taking vacations or time away from work. In conclusion, chronic stress can have a detrimental effect on brain function and contribute to brain fog. However, implementing strategies to reduce stress levels and promote relaxed states can help optimize brain health and minimize cognitive dysfunction.

Chapter 6: Coping Strategies for Brain Fog

Living with brain fog can be frustrating and overwhelming, but there are several coping strategies that can help you manage your symptoms and improve your cognitive function. In this chapter, we will explore some of the most effective coping strategies for brain fog.

SUBCHAPTER 6.1: LIFESTYLE CHANGES

One of the most important ways to cope with brain fog is to make lifestyle changes that promote brain health and reduce symptoms. Here are some lifestyle changes you can make:

Get Adequate Sleep

Sleep is essential for brain health, and getting enough sleep can help reduce brain fog symptoms. Try to establish a regular sleep schedule and get seven to nine hours of sleep each night.

Exercise Regularly

Exercise is not only good for your physical health, but also for your brain health. Regular exercise can improve cognitive function and reduce brain fog symptoms. Try to get at least 30 minutes of moderate exercise most days of the week.

Eat a Healthy Diet

Eating a healthy diet can provide your brain with the nutrients and energy it needs to function properly. Focus on eating whole foods, such as fruits, vegetables, whole grains, lean proteins, and healthy fats. Avoid processed and sugary foods, which can contribute to brain fog symptoms.

Reduce Stress

Stress can exacerbate brain fog symptoms, so it's important to find ways to manage stress. Try relaxation techniques, such as deep breathing, meditation, or yoga. Engage in activities that you enjoy and that help you relax, such as reading, listening to music, or taking a warm bath.

SUBCHAPTER 6.2: NUTRITIONAL SUPPLEMENTS

In addition to making lifestyle changes, there are several nutritional supplements that may help improve cognitive function and reduce brain fog symptoms. Here are some supplements to consider:

Omega-3 Fatty Acids

Omega-3 fatty acids are essential fats that have been linked to improved brain function. They can be found in fatty fish, such as salmon and sardines, as well as in fish oil supplements.

Vitamin B12

Vitamin B12 is important for brain function and is often deficient in people with brain fog symptoms. Consider taking a B12 supplement or eating more B12-rich foods, such as eggs, dairy, and meat.

Ginkgo Biloba

Ginkgo biloba is an herbal supplement that has been shown to improve cognitive function and reduce brain fog symptoms. It's available in supplement form and can be found at most health food stores.

SUBCHAPTER 6.3: MENTAL EXERCISES

Just as physical exercise can improve brain function, mental exercises can also help reduce brain fog symptoms. Here are some mental exercises to consider:

Puzzles and Games

Engaging in puzzles and games, such as crossword puzzles and Sudoku, can help improve cognitive function and reduce brain fog symptoms.

Memory Exercises

Memory exercises, such as memorizing lists or recalling past events, can help improve memory function and reduce brain fog symptoms.

Mindfulness Meditation

Mindfulness meditation involves focusing your attention on the present moment and can help reduce stress and improve cognitive function. Consider taking a mindfulness meditation class or using a guided meditation app. By making lifestyle changes, taking nutritional supplements, and engaging in mental exercises, you can cope with brain fog symptoms and improve your cognitive function. These coping strategies may take time and effort, but they can ultimately lead to a better quality of life.

SUBCHAPTER 6.1: LIFESTYLE CHANGES

When dealing with brain fog and cognitive dysfunction, lifestyle changes can play a vital role in the management and improvement of symptoms. Here are some lifestyle changes that may be helpful:

1. Exercise

When struggling with brain fog, it can be tough to find the motivation to exercise regularly. However, regular physical activity can be extremely helpful in reducing stress and improving overall cognitive function. Even simply going for a walk or doing some light stretching can make a big difference.

2. Sleep

Many people who experience brain fog also suffer from poor sleep quality. Improving sleep habits, such as going to bed and waking up at the same time each day, reducing caffeine intake, and creating a calming bedtime routine, can help to improve the quality and duration of sleep.

3. Nutrition

The food we eat can have a significant impact on cognitive function. Eating a balanced diet that is rich in fruits, vegetables, lean proteins, and healthy fats can help to improve mental clarity and reduce brain fog. Additionally, it is important to avoid processed foods, sugary drinks, and excess alcohol.

4. Stress Reduction

High levels of stress can exacerbate symptoms of brain fog. It is important to find healthy ways to manage stress, such as practicing mindfulness, yoga, meditation, or deep breathing exercises. Additionally, finding hobbies or activities that you enjoy can provide a much-needed mental break and reduce stress levels.

5. Avoiding Environmental Triggers

For many people, environmental triggers such as loud noises, bright lights, or strong scents can worsen brain fog symptoms. It is important to identify and avoid these triggers as much as possible. By implementing these lifestyle changes, individuals dealing with brain fog and cognitive dysfunction can help to manage their symptoms and improve their quality of life.

SUBCHAPTER 6.2: NUTRITIONAL SUPPLEMENTS

One approach to managing brain fog is taking nutritional supplements. Certain supplements have been shown to support brain function and potentially improve cognitive function. Omega-3 fatty acids, found in fish oil supplements, have been linked to improved memory and cognitive function. Vitamin B12 is also important for proper brain function, as it helps regulate the production of neurotransmitters. Additionally, vitamin D has been shown to play a role in mental health, as deficiencies have been linked to depression and dementia. Other supplements that may improve cognitive function include gingko biloba, which has been used for centuries as a memory aid, and acetyl-L-carnitine, which has been shown to improve focus and memory recall. It is important to note that supplements should be taken under the guidance of a healthcare professional, as some supplements may interact with certain medications or have adverse effects. Additionally, supplements should not be a replacement for a healthy and balanced diet. In conclusion, incorporating certain nutritional supplements into a balanced well-rounded diet may potentially improve brain function and cognitive health. However, it is important to consult with a healthcare professional before starting any supplement regimen.

Brain Fog: Coping with mental fatigue and cognitive dysfunction

SUBCHAPTER 6.3: MENTAL EXERCISES

Mental exercises are a vital part of managing brain fog. When practiced consistently, these exercises can help improve cognitive function and enhance mental clarity. Here are some of the best mental exercises that you can perform on a routine basis:

1. Meditation

Meditation is a great way to calm your mind and reduce stress. This technique involves focusing your attention on your breath or a certain object, and clearing your mind of all other thoughts. Consistent meditation has shown to improve attention and decrease anxiety.

2. Brain Training Apps

There are numerous brain-training apps available that can help improve working memory, attention, and problem-solving skills. These apps offer various exercises and games that work on different aspects of cognitive function.

3. Reading

Regular reading is an excellent way to keep your brain active and improve your cognitive function. Fictional stories and novels can stimulate your imagination and creativity, while non-fiction can teach you new skills and knowledge.

4. Puzzles and Games

Solving puzzles and playing games like crossword puzzles, Sudoku, and chess can help improve your memory and concentration. These activities also challenge your brain and stimulate your problem-solving skills.

5. Learning a New Skill

Learning a new skill or language is an excellent way to challenge your brain and improve cognitive function. This can be an instrument, a new language, or coding. It also enhances creative thinking and provides an outlet for personal growth. Performing these exercises regularly can help improve your mental clarity, enhance memory, and decrease brain fog. Consistency is key to reaping the benefits of these practices.

Chapter 7: Cognitive Rehabilitation

Cognitive rehabilitation is a set of techniques and therapies aimed at improving cognitive or thinking skills that have been lost or impaired due to a variety of reasons including injury, disease or aging. The main goal of cognitive rehabilitation is to help the individual regain independence and quality of life by improving their cognitive abilities.

TYPES OF COGNITIVE REHABILITATION

There are several types of cognitive rehabilitation, including computerized training, cognitive exercises, and group therapy. Computerized training involves using various computer programs designed to improve cognitive skills such as attention, memory, and problem-solving skills. Cognitive exercises involve practicing specific cognitive skills such as memory recall, attention to detail, and problem-solving. Group therapy involves working with other individuals who have similar cognitive problems and can provide mutual support and encouragement.

BENEFITS OF COGNITIVE REHABILITATION

Cognitive rehabilitation can help improve memory, attention, executive function, processing speed, and other cognitive abilities. It can also improve the ability to perform activities of daily living, social skills, and communication. Furthermore, cognitive rehabilitation can increase the level of independence and quality of life of the person receiving therapy.

WHO CAN BENEFIT FROM COGNITIVE REHABILITATION?

Cognitive rehabilitation is beneficial for individuals who have suffered from traumatic brain injury, stroke, dementia, or other neurological disorders that have caused cognitive dysfunction. It is also helpful for individuals who are aging and may experience mild cognitive impairment or normal age-related declines in cognitive functioning.

HOW DOES COGNITIVE REHABILITATION WORK?

Cognitive rehabilitation is tailored to the individual needs of the person receiving therapy. A cognitive assessment is conducted to evaluate the scope and severity of cognitive deficits. This assessment helps to identify the specific cognitive strengths and weaknesses of the individual and provides a basis for developing a personalized cognitive rehabilitation plan.

The Rehabilitation Plan

The rehabilitation plan is created based on the individual's specific needs, preferences, and goals. It may include exercises and activities aimed at improving attention, memory, processing speed, executive functioning, and problem-solving skills. The rehabilitation plan may also involve technology such as computer programs designed to improve cognitive skills.

Individual versus Group Therapy

Individual therapy provides more individualized attention and can focus specifically on an individual's unique needs. However, group therapy can offer additional benefits such as peer support and group accountability. A combination of individual and group therapy can provide a comprehensive approach to cognitive rehabilitation.

CONCLUSION

Cognitive rehabilitation can help improve cognitive abilities in individuals who have suffered from neurological disorders. It can be done through various techniques and is tailored to the specific needs and goals of the individual. Cognitive rehabilitation is a useful way to improve cognitive function and ultimately, quality of life.

Chapter 8: Medications for Brain Fog

If lifestyle changes, supplements, and cognitive rehabilitation do not work for you, medications might be a next step to consider. In general, medication should only be used when other methods fail, and only under the supervision of a doctor. There are many different medications that may be used to treat brain fog and cognitive dysfunction. Some of these include:

CHOLINESTERASE INHIBITORS:

These drugs work by increasing levels of acetylcholine, a neurotransmitter that is important for memory and learning. They are commonly used to treat Alzheimer's disease, but may also be helpful for brain fog caused by other conditions. Examples of cholinesterase inhibitors include donepezil, galantamine, and rivastigmine.

STIMULANTS:

Stimulants are commonly used to treat ADHD, but may also be helpful for brain fog caused by other conditions. These medications work by increasing the level of dopamine and norepinephrine in the brain, which can improve focus and concentration. Examples of stimulants used for brain fog include methylphenidate, amphetamines, and modafinil.

ANTIDEPRESSANTS:

Antidepressants may be helpful in treating brain fog caused by depression or anxiety. These medications work by altering levels of neurotransmitters such as serotonin and norepinephrine in the brain. Examples of antidepressants include selective serotonin reuptake inhibitors (SSRIs), such as fluoxetine and sertraline, and serotonin-norepinephrine reuptake inhibitors (SNRIs), such as duloxetine and venlafaxine.

B VITAMINS:

B vitamins are essential for brain health, and deficiencies in these vitamins have been linked to cognitive problems. Some people with brain fog may benefit from taking B vitamin supplements or injections.

Side Effects and Risks of Medications

All medications have potential side effects and risks, and it is important to discuss these with your doctor. Some common side effects of medications used to treat brain fog include nausea, dizziness, headache, and insomnia. In addition, some medications may interact with other medications or medical conditions, so it is important to inform your doctor of all medications and medical conditions you have.

Conclusion

Medication may be a helpful option for some people with brain fog, but it should not be the first line of treatment. Lifestyle changes, supplements, and cognitive rehabilitation should be tried first, under the guidance of a healthcare professional. When medication is prescribed, it should be closely monitored and only used as directed.

Chapter 9: Alternative Therapies to Improve Cognitive Function

When it comes to brain fog and cognitive dysfunction, there are a variety of alternative therapies that may help improve cognitive function. While not all of these therapies have been widely studied, some people have reported positive results from them. It is essential to note that it is always best to consult with a medical professional before starting any new therapy.

ACUPUNCTURE

Acupuncture is an ancient Chinese practice that involves inserting thin needles into specific points on the body. It is commonly used to treat pain, stress, and other conditions. Studies have shown that acupuncture may help improve cognitive function for people with brain fog and cognitive dysfunction. It is believed that acupuncture may help boost blood flow to the brain, which can improve cognitive function.

MEDITATION

Meditation is a relaxation technique that involves focusing on the present moment. It has been shown to reduce anxiety, stress, and depression. Some studies have suggested that meditation may help improve cognitive function. It is believed that meditation may help increase blood flow to the brain and reduce inflammation, both of which can improve cognitive function.

YOGA

Yoga is a mind-body practice that involves postures, breathing techniques, and meditation. It has been shown to reduce stress, anxiety, and depression. Some studies have suggested that yoga may help improve cognitive function. It is believed that yoga may help increase blood flow to the brain, reduce inflammation, and improve overall brain function.

CHIROPRACTIC CARE

Chiropractic care is a form of alternative medicine that involves the manipulation of the spine and other joints. It is commonly used to treat back pain, neck pain, and other musculoskeletal conditions. Some studies have suggested that chiropractic care may help improve cognitive function. It is believed that chiropractic adjustments may help increase blood flow to the brain and reduce inflammation, both of which can improve cognitive function.

AROMATHERAPY

Aromatherapy is a holistic healing practice that involves the use of essential oils. It is commonly used to reduce stress, anxiety, and depression. Some studies have suggested that aromatherapy may help improve cognitive function. It is believed that certain essential oils, such as rosemary and peppermint, may help improve memory and concentration.

CONCLUSION

Alternative therapies can be a valuable tool for those struggling with brain fog and cognitive dysfunction. While more research is needed to determine their effectiveness, many people have reported positive outcomes from using these therapies. However, it is crucial to note that these therapies should not replace traditional medical treatments and should be used in conjunction with medical care.

Chapter 10: Coping with Brain Fog at Work

Brain fog can significantly impact our ability to be productive and efficient at work. It can make daily tasks more challenging, increase stress levels, and lead to feelings of frustration and inadequacy. However, there are strategies that can be implemented to help cope with brain fog in the workplace.

UNDERSTANDING WORK-RELATED BRAIN FOG

Work-related brain fog is a type of cognitive dysfunction that can be triggered by various factors such as work-related stress, lack of sleep, dehydration, poor nutrition, and attempting to multitask. The symptoms of brain fog at work include difficulty concentrating, forgetfulness, slow thinking, difficulty processing information, and a reduced ability to problem-solve.

STRATEGIES FOR COPING WITH BRAIN FOG AT WORK

1. Prioritize: When experiencing brain fog, it's essential to prioritize tasks to ensure that

important work is completed first. This can help reduce stress levels and increase productivity. 2. Take breaks: It can be helpful to take frequent short breaks in order to rest and recharge the brain. It's important to physically step away from the work setting to fully disconnect from work-related tasks. 3. Improve nutrition: Eating a healthy, balanced diet can have a significant impact on brain function. Nutritious foods such as fruits, vegetables, and low-fat proteins can fuel the brain and reduce symptoms of brain fog. 4. Stay hydrated: Drinking water regularly throughout the workday is important for maintaining cognitive function. Dehydration can lead to symptoms of brain fog, so staying hydrated can help prevent this. 5. Reduce multitasking: Trying to do too many things at once can worsen symptoms of brain fog and decrease overall productivity. Instead, focus on one task at a time and complete it before moving onto the next. 6. Establish clear lines of communication: Communication is key in any work environment, but it becomes even more important when coping with brain fog. It can be helpful to be transparent with colleagues about what's happening and set clear expectations so that everyone is on the same page.

Additional Tips

• Use memory aids such as notes or lists to help remember important details. • Implement stress-reducing techniques such as deep breathing or meditation. • Limit caffeine and alcohol intake, as these can worsen symptoms of brain fog.

CONCLUSION

Managing brain fog in the workplace is important for maintaining productivity, reducing stress levels, and improving overall job satisfaction. By implementing the strategies outlined in this chapter, it's possible to effectively cope with work-related brain fog and achieve success in the workplace.

Chapter 11: Brain Fog and Relationships

Living with brain fog can be a challenge, and it can affect your social life, including friendships, romantic relationships, and parenting. Brain fog makes it difficult to focus and communicate properly, which can strain relationships with others. In this chapter, we will explore different types of relationships and discuss how to cope with brain fog while maintaining healthy relationships.

SUBCHAPTER 11.1: FRIENDSHIPS

Friendships are an essential part of a happy and healthy life. However, maintaining friendships can be challenging when you have brain fog. Symptoms such as forgetfulness and difficulty concentrating can make it difficult to hold a conversation or remember important details. It's important to communicate your struggles with your friends so they can understand and support you. Here are a few tips to help you maintain friendships despite brain fog:

Keep Your Friends Informed:

Let your friends know about your condition and how it affects your day-to-day life. This way, they won't assume that your forgetfulness or lack of focus is due to disinterest or negligence.

Choose Low-Stress Activities:

When hanging out with friends, choose low-stress activities that don't require a lot of mental or physical effort. A movie night or a relaxed dinner can be a great way to catch up without adding stress to your life.

Be Honest:

If you're feeling overwhelmed or struggling to focus during a conversation, be honest with your friends about how you're feeling. They will appreciate your honesty, and it will help them understand how to better support you.

SUBCHAPTER 11.2: ROMANTIC RELATIONSHIPS

Romantic relationships can be challenging for anyone, but living with brain fog can add extra stress. Symptoms such as fatigue and forgetfulness can be mistaken for lack of interest or emotional distance. It's important to communicate with your partner and work together to manage brain fog symptoms. Here are a few tips to help you navigate a romantic relationship while coping with brain fog:

Communicate Openly:

Be honest with your partner about your condition and how it affects your life. Having an open conversation about your struggles can help your partner understand your needs and offer support.

Find Low-Stress Activities to Do Together:

Choose low-stress activities that allow you to spend time together without adding extra stress to your life. Going for a walk or cooking dinner together can be great ways to connect without adding mental or physical strain.

Create Shared Systems:

Brain fog can make it difficult to remember important details or tasks. Work with your partner to create a shared calendar or to-do list to help you keep track of important dates and tasks.

SUBCHAPTER 11.3: PARENTING

Parenting can be challenging under the best of circumstances, but living with brain fog can make it even harder. Symptoms such as forgetfulness and difficulty concentrating can make it difficult to stay organized and keep up with the demands of parenting. Here are a few tips to help you manage parenting while coping with brain fog:

Keep a Routine:

Establishing a daily routine can help you stay organized and reduce stress. Try to wake up at the same time every day and create a schedule for meals, playtime, and naps.

Get Support:

Ask for help from family and friends when you need it. Having an extra set of hands to help with childcare or household tasks can be invaluable when you're feeling overwhelmed.

Be Kind to Yourself:

Parenting is hard work, and it's important to be kind to yourself. Remember that brain fog is a real condition that can affect your abilities. Don't beat yourself up for making mistakes or needing extra help.

CONCLUSION

Brain fog can make maintaining healthy relationships a challenge. However, with open communication and a few coping strategies, you can continue to build and maintain meaningful relationships with friends, partners, and children. It's important to remember that brain fog is a real condition that affects many people, and there is no shame in needing extra support.

SUBCHAPTER 11.1: FRIENDSHIPS

Living with brain fog can be a challenge, and it can greatly affect your social life. Maintaining friendships may seem difficult due to the symptoms of Brain Fog, but it's essential to keep your social relationships intact to avoid the isolation that comes with this condition. One of the most critical aspects of maintaining friendships with brain fog is communication. Your friends may not fully understand the symptoms of brain fog unless you explain them. Educating your friends on your condition helps them become more understanding and supportive. Another critical factor is being honest with your friends about what you can and cannot do. You may need to cancel plans at the last minute, and your friend may feel frustrated, but explaining why you cannot attend will help them understand. It's also fundamental to find friends who are compassionate and understanding.

Surrounding yourself with positive people who support and accept you for who you are will positively influence your mental state. Look for people who are patient and can support you through the tough times. Managing your time and energy levels is another important aspect of maintaining friendships with brain fog. You may need to limit the amount of time you spend with your friends, but that doesn't mean you should eliminate socializing entirely. Try setting up shorter meetings or communicating via phone or text to stay in touch with your friends without over-exerting yourself. In conclusion, maintaining friendships with brain fog can be challenging but not impossible. Communication, honesty, finding understanding friends, and managing time and energy levels are crucial to keep social relationships thriving. Don't be afraid to reach out and ask for support when you need it. Remember, strong friendships are loyal, supportive, and understanding, and you deserve to have them in your life.

SUBCHAPTER 11.2: ROMANTIC RELATIONSHIPS

Living with brain fog can take a toll on your romantic relationships. It can be difficult to maintain a healthy and strong relationship with your partner when you are struggling with cognitive dysfunction. Here are some tips on how to cope with brain fog in your romantic relationships:

Communicate with your partner

It's important to communicate with your partner about your struggles with brain fog. Let them know how it affects you and your relationship, and how they can help support you. Be open and honest, and try to find ways to work together to overcome these challenges.

Be patient with yourself and your partner

Dealing with brain fog can be frustrating, but it's important to be patient with yourself and your partner. Remember that you are both doing the best you can, and that it may take time to find the right strategies to cope with cognitive dysfunction.

Find new ways to connect

When brain fog makes it difficult to engage in your usual activities with your partner, try to find new and alternative ways to connect. For example, if your usual date night involves a lot of conversation, try watching a movie together instead. You can still enjoy each other's company without having to strain your cognitive abilities.

Consider couples therapy

Couples therapy can be a helpful way to work through the challenges of living with brain fog in a romantic relationship. A therapist can help you and your partner communicate effectively, develop coping strategies, and strengthen your bond. Remember, living with brain fog does not mean you cannot have a healthy and fulfilling romantic relationship. With patience, communication, and a willingness to try new things, you can overcome these challenges and build a stronger connection with your partner.

CHAPTER 11.3: BRAIN FOG AND PARENTING

Parenting can be challenging even at the best of times, but when brain fog strikes, it can feel like an insurmountable obstacle. For many parents who experience brain fog, the condition can leave them feeling guilty, frustrated, and overwhelmed, which can make it difficult to be present and attentive to their children. In this subchapter, we'll explore some strategies for making parenting with brain fog a little bit easier.

Be Kind to Yourself

One of the most important things you can do when parenting with brain fog is to be kind to yourself. Acknowledge that brain fog is a real condition that affects your ability to think clearly and focus, and that it's not your fault. Give yourself permission to take breaks when you need them, and don't beat yourself up for not being able to do everything on your to-do list. Remember that taking care of yourself is essential for taking care of your children.

Set Realistic Expectations

When you're experiencing brain fog, it's essential to set realistic expectations for yourself and your children. This may mean scaling back on your usual routines and expectations until you have more energy and mental clarity. Focus on the things that are most important, such as spending quality time with your children and making sure they are safe and healthy. Don't be afraid to ask for help from family and friends when you need it.

Plan Ahead

One way to make parenting with brain fog a little easier is to plan ahead as much as possible. This means creating routines and systems that work for your family, and being prepared for unexpected events. Make lists of tasks that need to be done, and prioritize them according to importance. Consider using tools such as calendars, reminders, and alarms to help you stay on track.

Be Open with Your Children

Finally, it's important to be open with your children about your condition. Depending on their age, you can explain to them that you may have trouble concentrating or remembering things sometimes, but that it's not their fault. Encourage them to ask questions and express their feelings, and let them know that you are always there for them, even when you're feeling foggy. In conclusion, parenting with brain fog can be challenging, but it's important to remember that you're not alone. By being kind to yourself, setting realistic expectations, planning ahead, and being open with your children, you can make the experience a little bit easier. Remember that taking care of yourself is essential for taking care of your children, and that there are resources available to help you cope with brain fog.

Chapter 12: When to Seek Professional Help

If you have been experiencing brain fog symptoms for a prolonged period of time and your daily life is being significantly affected, it may be time to seek professional help. While lifestyle modifications like exercise, nutrition, and mental exercises can be helpful for brain fog, they may not be enough in all cases. There are several healthcare professionals who can be consulted to help manage brain fog. Some options include neurologists, psychiatrists, psychologists, and cognitive behavioral therapists. These professionals are all trained to assess and manage cognitive dysfunction like brain fog. If you decide to seek professional help, you will likely be assessed through cognitive testing. This testing typically includes tasks like memory testing, attention and focus testing, and reaction time testing. This is done to evaluate your cognitive function and help identify the root of your brain fog symptoms. Treatment options may include prescription medication, cognitive rehabilitation, therapy, and/or lifestyle modifications. Your healthcare professional may also recommend additional testing such as imaging or bloodwork to rule out other health conditions that may be contributing to your brain fog. It's important to remember that it's okay to seek help. Brain fog can be frustrating and may interfere with your daily life. Seeking professional help can help you gain control over your cognitive dysfunction and help you feel like yourself again.

When to seek emergency care

While brain fog symptoms can be concerning, they may not always warrant an emergency room visit. However, certain symptoms may indicate a medical emergency. If you experience sudden and severe confusion, trouble speaking, weakness on one side of your body, or sudden changes in vision, seek immediate medical attention. These symptoms could indicate a stroke or other serious medical condition that requires immediate treatment. It's important to be aware of your symptoms and seek professional help when needed. With the right treatment plan, it's possible to manage brain fog and regain control over your daily life.

Chapter 13: Dealing with the Emotional Impact of Brain Fog

Living with brain fog can be a challenging experience, both physically and emotionally. For those affected by it, the feeling of being unable to think clearly or remember things can be incredibly frustrating and even distressing. In addition to these directly observable effects, brain fog can also have an emotional impact on individuals that is not always immediately apparent.

EMOTIONAL IMPACT OF BRAIN FOG

One of the most common emotional effects of brain fog is the sense of frustration or helplessness that it can create. When a person's cognitive abilities are impaired, they may find it difficult to complete tasks or remember important information. This can make them feel overwhelmed and powerless, leading to feelings of anxiety or depression. Another potential emotional effect of brain fog is a sense of isolation or social withdrawal. When it becomes challenging to keep up with conversations or engage in social activities, people may start to feel as if they are losing touch with the world around them. This can lead to feelings of loneliness or even social anxiety. Finally, brain fog can also impact a person's self-esteem. When they find it difficult to perform tasks or remember things that they could previously do with ease, they may begin to doubt their abilities. This can lead to a sense of low self-worth or even shame.

STRATEGIES TO COPE WITH THE EMOTIONAL EFFECTS OF BRAIN FOG

While dealing with the emotional impact of brain fog can be challenging, there are a variety of strategies that can help individuals to manage these feelings. Here are some effective coping strategies that may be helpful:

Practice Self-Compassion

The first step to coping with the emotional impact of brain fog is to acknowledge that these feelings are normal and valid. Be kind to yourself and give yourself permission to feel frustrated or anxious. Don't beat yourself up for experiencing these emotions – instead, try to practice self-compassion and treat yourself with kindness.

Stay Connected with Others

One of the most damaging effects of brain fog is social isolation and withdrawal. Staying connected with others can help to combat these feelings. Make an effort to attend social events or meet up with friends on a regular basis, even if it takes extra effort to focus on what is being said.

Cultivate a Support System

Having a support system in place can be incredibly helpful when dealing with the emotional effects of brain fog. Talk to close friends or family members about how you are feeling and let them know what they can do to support you. Consider joining a support group where you can connect with others who are experiencing similar challenges.

Seek Professional Help

If you are struggling with depression, anxiety, or other emotional effects of brain fog, it may be helpful to seek professional help. A therapist or counselor can provide support and guidance as you navigate the challenges of this condition.

Find Ways to Boost Your Confidence

If brain fog is impacting your self-esteem, find ways to boost your confidence and sense of self-worth. This could involve taking on a new challenge or hobby, learning a new skill, or simply taking time to practice self-care and do things that you enjoy.

CONCLUSION

Dealing with the emotional impact of brain fog can be a challenge, but it is possible to manage these feelings and maintain a positive outlook. By practicing self-compassion, staying connected with others, seeking professional help when needed, and finding ways to boost your confidence, you can cope with the emotional effects of brain fog and live a fulfilling life.

Chapter 14: Future of Brain Fog Research

Brain fog is a little-understood condition that affects a significant number of people. For many, it can be a debilitating and frustrating experience that can impact their ability to live life to the fullest. Thankfully, researchers around the world are working tirelessly to unravel the mysteries of brain fog in the hopes of developing more effective treatments.

CURRENT STATE OF BRAIN FOG RESEARCH

Researchers are making progress in understanding brain fog and its underlying causes. Recent studies have focused on:

Neuroinflammation

Inflammation within the brain can cause brain fog. This inflammation can be caused by a range of factors, including viral and bacterial infections, stress, and autoimmune disorders. Researchers are exploring new treatments to reduce neuroinflammation and reduce brain fog symptoms.

Gut-Brain Axis

Emerging research suggests a strong link between the gut microbiome and brain function. It appears that the bacteria in our gut can influence brain function and contribute to brain fog. Researchers are working to gain a better understanding of this connection, with the hope of developing new therapies to help manage brain fog.

Hormonal Imbalances

Hormonal imbalances can lead to brain fog, particularly in women going through menopause or those with thyroid imbalances. Researchers are studying how hormone levels impact brain fog and exploring new treatments to help manage hormonal imbalances.

FUTURE DIRECTIONS OF BRAIN FOG RESEARCH

The future of brain fog research looks promising. New developments on the horizon include:

Gene Therapy

Researchers are exploring gene therapy approaches to brain fog treatment. These approaches could provide a patient-specific treatment, addressing the specific underlying causes of brain fog on a genetic level.

Personalized Medicine

As researchers gain a deeper understanding of the underlying causes of brain fog, personalized medicine approaches are expected to emerge. These approaches will allow healthcare providers to tailor treatments to the unique needs of each patient.

Artificial Intelligence

Artificial intelligence is expected to play a significant role in the future of brain fog research. By processing vast amounts of data, AI systems could help identify new patterns and connections that may not be visible to human researchers.

CONCLUSION

The future of brain fog research looks bright. While there is still much to learn about this complex condition, researchers are making significant progress in understanding the underlying causes of brain fog. With new technologies and approaches emerging, the hope is that we will see more effective treatments for brain fog in the near future.